# HOLISTIC HEALTH
## AND THE NEW
## MEDICINE

## John Ankerberg
## & John Weldon

HARVEST HOUSE PUBLISHERS
Eugene, Oregon 97402

### Other books by
### John Ankerberg
### and John Weldon

*The Facts on Astrology*
*The Facts on the New Age Movement*
*The Facts on Spirit Guides*
*The Facts on the Masonic Lodge*
*The Facts on the Jehovah's Witnesses*
*The Facts on the Mormon Church*
*The Facts on False Teaching in the Church*
*The Facts on Hinduism in America*
*The Facts on the Occult*
*The Facts on Islam*
*The Facts on Rock Music*

**THE FACTS ON HOLISTIC HEALTH AND
THE NEW MEDICINE**

Copyright © 1992 by The Ankerberg
  Theological Research Institute
Published by Harvest House Publishers
Eugene, Oregon 97402

ISBN 0-89081-973-4

# *CONTENTS*

## SECTION ONE
## Introduction to the New Medicine

1. Why is the subject of holistic health
   and the new medicine important? .............. 5

## SECTION TWO
## Specific Practices and Treatments
## of the New Medicine

2. What are acupuncture and acupressure? .......... 8

3. What are altered states of consciousness? ......... 9

4. What is anthroposophical medicine? ............ 10

5. What is attitudinal healing? .................... 10

6. What is autogenic training? .................... 11

7. What is Ayurvedic medicine? ................... 11

8. What are bioenergetics (neo-
   Reichian bodywork) and Reichian
   therapy (orgonomy)? ......................... 12

9. What is biofeedback? .......................... 13

10. What are bodywork methods? ................. 14

11. What is breath awareness? ..................... 15

12. What is (medical) channeling? ................. 16

13. What is chiropractic? ......................... 17

14. What is chromotherapy/color therapy? ......... 21

15. What is crystal healing/crystal work? .......... 22

16. What is dowsing, water dowsing? .............. 23

17. What is dream work? ......................... 24

18. What are the Edgar Cayce methods of healing? . 25

19. What is herbal medicine? ...................... 26

20. What is homeopathy? ......................... 27

21. What are hypnosis and hypnotic regression? .... 28

22. What is (New Age) intuition? .................. 30

23. What is iridology? ............................ 31

24. What is Kirlian photography? ................. 32

25. What are the martial arts? .................... 33

26. What is (New Age) meditation? ................ 34

27. What is muscle testing? ....................... 35

28. What is naturopathy? .......................... 36

29. What is osteopathy? ........................... 37

30. What is polarity therapy? ..................... 38

31. What are psychic anatomies? .................. 38

32. What are psychic diagnosis, psychic
    healing, and psychic surgery? ............... 39

33. What is (medical) psychometry (radionics)? ..... 39

34. What is psychosynthesis? ...................... 40

35. What is reflexology? .......................... 41

36. What is Reiki? ................................ 41

37. What is self-help therapy? ..................... 42

38. What is shamanistic medicine? ................ 42

39. What is subliminal programming? ............ 43

40. What is therapeutic touch? .................... 44

41. What is Touch for Health? .................... 45

42. What is visualization? ........................ 45

43. What is yoga? ................................. 46

    Conclusion

    Recommended Reading

# SECTION ONE

## Introduction to the New Medicine

### 1. Why is the subject of holistic health and the New Medicine important?

Literally tens of millions of people in the Western world have been exposed to or use holistic* health methods. The occult revival and discontent over traditional medical care, sometimes justified, has opened the door to a wide variety of alternate therapies in society. Indeed, *Time* (Nov. 4, 1991) reported that alternate medicine is "now a 27 *billion*-a-year industry," noting that 30 percent of those polled had tried an unconventional therapy. According to *Medical World News* (May 11, 1987), the overall cost of suspected health-care fraud is approaching $30 *billion* annually. Promoters of holistic health techniques and the New Medicine prosper by offering patients simple solutions to complex diseases as well as practices and remedies that are said to be free of side effects. Today, even thousands of medical doctors and nurses use these methods.

We certainly have no quarrel with any medical method whose safety and efficacy has been established. Our concern is with the widespread promotion of methods which have either not been proven, or are questionable on other (physical or spiritual) grounds.

While we do not minimize the problems of conventional medical treatment, our research shows that the holistic health movement as a whole is largely based upon ineffective and/or potentially dangerous methods that are not in the best interest of the patient. By and large, holistic methods reject what is known about how the human body works and are generally opposed to a scientific approach to health care.

When the New Medicine claims to "work," it works for none of the reasons characteristically cited by its promoters. Things *can* work and still be dangerous, such as car

---

* claiming to treat the "whole" person, body, mind and spirit

5

bombs. Things can work and still be both wrong and dangerous, such as practices that rely upon occultic methods. Finally, things can be false and only *seem* to work. Innumerable holistic treatments may at first appear to work on the basis of their claimed principles, but in reality work only for reasons relating to human psychology (the placebo effect) or time (the natural healing ability of the body).

Many holistic health practitioners have wrongly assumed that their treatments are effective based on misperceptions of empirical medicine (experience alone) rather than careful scientific testing. Given the variable nature of the disease process itself, virtually any holistic health treatment can boast a significant number of "success" stories, even in serious disease.

It is therefore vital to determine (1) whether or not a given procedure works on the basis of its stated principles, (2) the relative credibility of those principles, and (3) the true reason for its effectiveness when a method is effective. If something works or seems to work, it is vital to know why it works. Failing to answer that question can be costly.

Another serious concern is that occultism and spiritistic influence are frequently the source of power behind the origin and/or treatments of numerous specific holistic health practices. In addition to their lack of scientific credibility, these practices should be questioned because of their involvement with occult methods the Bible warns against (Deuteronomy 18:10-12). Occult powers may indeed heal a person physically (at least temporarily) but only at a much greater cost spiritually and psychologically.

Related to its occultic nature, holistic health methods are frequently found to depend upon some form of "energy" channeling. Many of these treatments claim to "balance" or "restore" or otherwise manipulate alleged invisible energies which supposedly exist or circulate within the human body. These energies are frequently associated with the mystical energies of occultic religion; e.g., the Hindu *prana*, Taoist *chi*, shamanistic *mana*, etc. Proponents claim that the real cause of illness and disease is an alleged disorder of this energy's "natural flow" and that unless the flow is properly restored, health cannot be maintained. In other words, in most of the New Medicine, the manipulation of occult energies and health care are inseparable. Unfortunately this manipulation of mystical energy is often an open door to spiritism under another name. It is difficult, if not impossible, to distinguish the use of "energy" manipulation and transference in many holistic health treatments from the manipulation of "energy" found among occultists in their various practices.

Holistic health therapists incorrectly interpret this energy as a *natural* or *divine* energy bringing physical and spiritual health when, in fact, it is an occultic, spiritistic energy detrimental to physical and spiritual health. We freely concede that "energy balancers" might be doing nothing at all, but involvement with genuine occultic powers cannot be ruled out.

In sum, because they are ineffective, holistic health treatments are potentially dangerous because they may fail to diagnose physical symptoms properly and thus never uncover a serious underlying condition that may progress toward further injury or death. It is always possible that an unconventional method of treatment may prove useful or suggest fruitful avenues for additional research. But before any method is widely accepted by the public, common sense teaches that its claims should be substantiated.

In addition, the New Medicine may be physically, psychologically, and/or spiritually consequential because to the extent its methods may lead a person into occult involvement it brings the same kinds of physical, psychological, and spiritual dangers associated with occult practices. Unfortunately, the response to coauthor John Weldon's two previous texts on this subject reveal that not only are holistic health methods increasingly employed by Christians, but even that many don't seem to care about the spiritual issues involved—as long as a practice "works." Too many people have unrealistic expectations concerning modern medicine—they almost expect miracles. But despite its great advances, scientific medicine is not perfect. However, to turn to occult medicine will only compound the problem at all levels.

In the following pages we briefly describe over 50 contemporary holistic health methods and/or adjuncts to treatment. While a few of these may be physically and spiritually neutral both safety and effectiveness must first be established before they can be recommended. Documentation for our conclusions relative to 12 of these subjects can be found in *Can You Trust Your Doctor?: The Complete Guide to New Age Medicine and Its Threat to Your Family* (Brentwood, TN: Wolgemuth & Hyatt, 1990). Documentation for all others is on file at The Ankerberg Theological Research Institute, Chattanooga, Tennessee in *New Age Medicine*, an unpublished manuscript of 1650 pages (4000 notes, 1100 bibliographic citations). Those desiring additional information on other therapies are urged to contact The National Council Against Health Fraud (see Recommended Reading).

# SECTION TWO

## *Specific Practices and Treatments of the New Medicine*

### 2. What are acupuncture and acupressure?

Acupuncture and acupressure are methods of applying stimulation to specific points on the body. Based on the occultic religion of Taoism, they claim to be able to stimulate the flow of cosmic life-energy known as *ki* (Japanese) or *chi* (Chinese) through alleged invisible channels or "meridians" in the body. When body organs or systems are supposedly deficient in a proper supply of *ki* or *chi* energy, imbalance is allegedly produced, resulting in disease. Restoring the flow of psychic energy through the meridians is believed to revitalize the body organs and systems, thereby curing illness and maintaining health.

Some scientists have claimed that acupuncture is effective for certain ailments and that it works on the basis of as yet unknown principles. But the latest scientific research is not supportive; studies have yet to demonstrate acupuncture's effectiveness. For example, an exhaustive analysis of research conducted to date published in *The Clinical Journal of Pain* (June 1991) concluded that acupuncture was at best a powerful placebo (cf. *Journal of Clinical Epidemiology*, 1990, Vol. 43, pp. 1191-99). When Western scientists attempt to separate acupuncture from its underlying occultic philosophy or practice and merely engage in an unspecific needle stimulation, these methods tend to lose their efficacy.

While the minority of scientific practitioners of acupuncture avoid the occult, most traditional practitioners do not. Classical acupuncture and acupressure involve the practice of an ancient pagan medicine inseparably tied to Taoism. In addition, Eastern meditative programs or other occultic practices may be used in conjunction with acupuncture therapy. Further, psychic healing may be deliberately or inadvertently engaged through the practice of attempting to regulate or channel psychic energies (see Question 32).

Needle stimulation has produced physical complications, such as infection and nerve damage. Infrequent serious injuries, such as punctured lung and convulsion, have also been reported: The complication frequency is unknown because no study has been done. Because diagnosis and treatment can be ineffective, the possibility of misdiagnosis of a serious illness also exists.

### 3. What are altered states of consciousness?

Writing in the *Journal of Transpersonal Psychology* (1974, No. 2, p. 125) psychologist and New Age consciousness researcher Kenneth Ring of the University of Connecticut observed that no period in Western psychology "has exceeded the present one in the interest taken in manipulating states of consciousness." In fact, there is a new global quest for cultivating altered consciousness reinforced by the fact that of some 4,000 modern societies, almost 90 percent already have procedures institutionalized for just such practices.

Altered states of consciousness are a product of the deliberate cultivation of abnormal states of consciousness—states not normally experienced apart from a specific technique or program (usually occultic), used to develop them. Millions of proponents claim that altered states allegedly produce a "higher" state of consciousness or "being," including dramatic spiritistic (occultic) revelations, psychic powers, personality alteration, and a "positive" restructuring of the participant's worldview along Eastern/occultic lines. Altered states are used for psychic diagnosis and psychic healing, and are frequently encountered as part of meditation programs which accompany many New Age therapies.

Scientific research in this area is a mixture of investigating normal, marginally altered consciousness (e.g., dreams) and occultic and parapsychological exploration of mystical, occultic states.

Cultivating altered states can be dangerous both emotionally and spiritually. Many cases of temporary and permanent insanity, spirit contact, occult transformation, and spirit possession have resulted. Incredibly, the temporary insanity is frequently interpreted as an indication of spiritual "enlightenment." Even spirit-possession itself is increasingly interpreted as an altered state of consciousness—allegedly a more evolved condition of existence. For further study, the research of Tal Brooke in *Riders of the Cosmic Circuit* is illustrative in the area of Eastern (Hindu) religious practice. The fact that altered states are routinely cultivated in meditation, dream work, shamanism, channeling, visualization, hypnosis, various self-help therapies, yoga, and many other practices indicates that they are widespread in society and responsible for a growing number of people being subjected to emotional damage or occult bondage.

## 4. What is anthroposophical medicine?

Anthroposophical medicine is an occult medicine based upon the philosophy of anthroposophy developed by necromancer Rudolph Steiner (1861–1925). It variously incorporates a belief in reincarnation, magic, astrology, animism, spiritism, and pantheism. Anthroposophical medicine claims to work by treating patients "spiritually" (occultly) not just phsyically. For example, by including concerns relative to patients' alleged past lives (health problems supposedly related to *karma*) and "spiritual" issues of their present life, anthroposophical doctors believe they can offer patients a more comprehensive "holistic" approach to health.

Even though over 1000 medical doctors employ it in their practice, anthroposophical medical theories and methods are based upon largely questionable, false, or occultic concepts which incorporate dubious medical theories of diagnosis and treatment. Patients run the risk of false diagnosis, occult treatments, or conversion to occultism.

## 5. What is attitudinal healing?

Attitudinal healing is an important component of the New Medicine that in various forms is practiced by millions of people. It involves the alleged regulation or maintenance of physical, mental, and/or spiritual health by learning supposedly "proper" (i.e., occultic) mental attitudes.

Attitudinal healing claims to work because the spirit, mind, and body are interrelated; therefore, proper mental attitudes may influence the entire person toward desired physical, psychological, and/or spiritual goals.

Although the health claims of New Age attitudinal healing have never been demonstrated, their occultic potential is clear; the common forms of practice are typically occultic, incorporating New Age philosophy and spiritistic revelations and contacts.

Occult texts frequently promote attitudinal healing. Medium Jane Robert's spirit guide endorses it in *The Nature of Personal Reality: A Seth Book.* The popular New Age bible called *A Course in Miracles* is also supportive. Both of these books are constituted from spiritistic revelations that were admittedly produced by occult means which the Bible forbids (Deuteronomy 18:9-12). These texts forcefully reject biblical teaching and promote occult philosophy and practice.

The danger of attitudinal healing is found in the adoption of occult philosophy and practice in the mistaken assumption it will bring physical, mental, and spiritual "health."

## 6. What is autogenic training?

Autogenic training is a medical "mind-body" therapy developed by psychiatrist J.H. Schulz and his student, Wolfgang Luth. It is the result, in part, of Schulz's observations of the hypnosis research of brain physiologist Oskar Vogt plus Schulz's own studies into yoga, Zen Buddhism, and hypnosis. The practice involves an eight-to-ten-week course that includes one hour per week of instruction plus various exercises three times a day. These exercises are designed to lead participants into a very deep state of relaxation. Visualization and meditation may also be employed (see Question 26,42).

Here, there is little difference between autogenic training and other self-hypnosis/meditation/visualization programs that may produce health benefits from nothing more than positive thinking and a relaxed mind and body. That many physical conditions will respond in some degree to a more relaxed lifestyle is not surprising. But these methods are far from cure-alls, and they may also have spiritual consequences more costly than their health benefits.

What is often not recognized in such practices is the occult potential and/or spiritual implications. For example, many methods of autogenic training are similar to those found in the psychosynthesis program developed by occultist Robert Assagioli (see Question 34). Techniques which employ hypnosis, New Age meditation, and visualization, and rely upon an alleged "inner self" for guidance have too many potential or actual associations with the occult.

## 7. What is Ayurvedic medicine?

Ayurvedic medicine is based on a Hindu approach to both the body and life in general. Its reliance upon Hinduism, an occultic religion, is what makes it attractive to many New Age therapists.

Ayurvedic medicine allegedly originated through revelations from the Hindu gods. Its concern is not merely physical health, but also maintaining mental and spiritual health as defined by Hinduism. Thus, Ayurvedic medicine is a spiritual method (the development of spiritual life according to Hindu beliefs) which incorporates physical concerns.

Ayurvedic medicine is not based upon traditional anatomy, but rather the spiritual (occult) anatomy of Hinduism (e.g., *chakras*. See Question 31). Because the ancient Indian physicians were also metaphysicians and because Hinduism teaches that the body is created out of consciousness, the medicine of Hinduism is a "medicine" of consciousness. Thus, looking at the "anatomical" charts of Ayurvedic medicine, one does not see the typical organs pictured in *Gray's Anatomy*, but rather a diagram of where the mind's consciousness is flowing as it "creates" the body. It is this alleged "psychic flow" that Ayurvedic medicine attempts to treat. This is why the Ayurvedic doctor does not merely treat the body, but also the more important mind/spirit.

Because each physical symptom is allegedly under the regulation of consciousness and/or the psychic energy flow known as *prana*, the goal is to modify the consciousness to cure the disease. In essence then, Ayurvedic medicine is the application of the occultic philosophy and practice of Hinduism (e.g., Brahman realization through yoga meditation) to medical practice.

Dr. Deepak Chopra is a practicing endocrinologist, former chief of staff of New England Memorial Medical Hospital in Stoneham, Maine, and founding president of the American Association of Ayurvedic Medicine. His *Quantum Healing: Exploring the Frontiers of Mind/Body Medicine*, along with Chandrashekhar G. Thakkur's *Ayurveda: The Indian Art and Science of Medicine*, and Baba Haridas and Dharma Sara Satsang's *Ayurveda: The Yoga of Health* clearly demonstrate the metaphysical and occultic nature of Ayruvedic medicine.

Thus, whatever else he practices, the Ayurvedic doctor practices an occultic religion which requires that his patients make an inner journey into the depths of Hinduism.

## 8. What are bioenergetics (neo-Reichian bodywork) and Reichian therapy (orgonomy)?

Bioenergetics or neo-Reichian bodywork was developed by Alexander Lowen, a disciplie of Wilhelm Reich's *Orgonomy* or *Reichian Therapy*. Reich (1897–1957), who dabbled in the occult, wrongly believed that the cause of many physical and mental disorders and illnesses was the inability to achieve a satisfactory orgasm. Thus, supposed sexual disfunction helps produce "character armor" and a psychological-physical response to the stresses of the outside world. Character armor could allegedly be loosened through "full orgastic gratification." In other words, Reich believed that for a patient to be cured he must be able to achieve gratification in the sexual act. He was convinced that blocking of sexual "bioenergy," which he called "orgone," was due to armoring—a condition that results from energy being bound in a muscular contraction and not being allowed to flow through the body. Reich proceeded to explore the therapeutic use of so-called orgone energy, which he also believed was the alleged "life energy" of the universe. In this sense, orgone is similar to other mystical energy concepts within New Age medicine such as *prana* and *chi*.

While Reich attempted to demonstrate both the reality and healing powers of this orgone energy, Alexander Lowen, a committed student, revised Reich's theories in accordance with his own findings. Rejecting the theory of orgone, he still accepted the concept behind it of a "life force" based upon mystical energy. Thus "bioenergetics" or neo-Reichian therapy involves the study of the human personality in terms of the alleged energetic processes of the body.

Bioenergetic therapy has two aspects. The first part involves the physical bodywork—bioenergetic exercises—in which the individual assumes yoga-like postures and performs breathing exercises in order to allegedly help relieve muscular tension which is obstructing the flow of energy.

Second, bioenergetic therapy utilizes counseling to discuss and analyze the individual's feelings before or after he has been treated. Bioenergetic is also based upon helping an individual to expand his mental consciousness by supposedly increasing his body consciousness. It attempts to go beyond both mechanical and mystical consciousness to unify mind and body consciousness toward more "awareness." The goal is to expand consciousness downward bringing a person closer to the "unconscious" in order to produce a new heightened consciousness of the unity and purpose of life. Nevertheless, these bodywork methods can also produce mystical experiences, and many patients seem to have some kind of transcendental experience in the course of therapy.

The effectiveness of bioenergetics has never been established and these therapies may encourage a client toward occult pursuits (see Question 10).

## 9. What is biofeedback?

Biofeedback is the use of special electronic equipment and mental exercises to influence physiological responses.

The goal is to gain some degree of control over particular physical functions that people do not normally, consciously regulate.

Mental control over bodily functions extends into antiquity through yoga and related practices. Elmer Green and Barbara Brown are among the most recognized modern leaders and innovators in biofeedback, although aspects of biofeedback principles and application were explored by earlier pioneers such as Johannes Schultz, the developer of autogenic training (see Question 6).

Biofeedback claims to work by enabling people to learn to recognize and consciously control certain biological parameters such as skin temperature, muscle tension, brain waves, pulse rate, etc. As a result, a person can better regulate physical problems normally associated with these parameters, such as tension headache, high blood pressure, etc.

Biofeedback offers only limited effectiveness for people who are highly motivated, and in particular, for those who are adept at visualization or meditation. Biofeedback can also be used to develop altered states of consciousness, psychic abilities, and spirit contact. In addition, it may offer unknown or unexpected consequences relating to manipulation of the consciousness.

While biofeedback is permissible in theory, we do not necessarily recommend the practice. As in hypnosis, unanswered questions remain, certain issues are tentative, and much work is experimental. Further, physical or mental problems may arise from improper use by unqualified therapists. Those people who choose to use biofeedback should avoid any occultic methods or applications and be certain of their practitioner's orientation and qualifications.

## 10. What are bodywork methods?

Bodywork methods, also known as the somatic sciences (e.g., rolfing, functional integration, orgonomy, bioenergetics, the Alexander method, and Arica) represent diverse methods both in practice and philosophy. Collectively they are used by millions of people. Frequently in these methods the body is used as a tool to help "enlighten" or otherwise influence the mind. The purpose is to supposedly improve mind-body functioning along a predetermined path or perspective that is in harmony with the underlying philosophy and goals of the particular bodywork method—goals which are often Eastern. This Eastern emphasis is documented in texts such as New Medicine authority Dr. Ken Dychtwald's *Bodymind*.

The influence of Wilhelm Reich (see Question 8) is seen in many bodywork methods, and similarities to yoga, an original bodywork technique, are frequently found. Because the body is usually believed to be a crude layer of mind, "proper" manipulation of the body may be used to impact the mind toward desired religious, psychological, or occultic goals.

Scientific testing is sparse although initial research and other considerations suggest that most of these methods do not work on the basis of their stated principles. For example, award-winning medical writer Hank Pizer's *Guide to the New Medicine: What Works, What Doesn't* (1982, p. 90) asserts, "There is little scientific evidence to support either the theoretical formulations on clinical effectiveness of either Rolfing or Feldenkrais [functional integration]." This is not to say they cannot have dramatic effects on a person's consciousness; they can. This is why many body-work methods are used in conjunction with various New Age therapies to help secure New Age goals, such as psychic development, yogic kundalini arousal, development of alleged "higher" consciousness, etc.

The problem with bodywork discipline is that most of its methods are clinically unevaluated and/or suspect in terms of the claims made. Many have occultic potential such as the dangerous phenomenon of yogic *kundalini* arousal—which seems to be a not infrequent occurrence in many bodywork methods (see Question 43). Further, the New Age religious philosophies underlying many of these methods can condition practitioners along New Age lines.

## 11. What is breath awareness?

A significant number of religions and psychotherapies employ "proper breathing" techniques as a supposed regulator of physical and psychological health, or for purposes of so-called spiritual (occult) enlightenment. Because breath awareness methods are often influenced by Eastern or occultic philosophy and practice (e.g., yoga) and because they are frequently designed to alter one's consciousness, they are also encountered in the many occultic forms of transpersonal and fringe psychotherapy. Eastern mystics and yogis have long claimed that the breath is a vital tool for altering one's consciousness. Concentration on the breath and regulation of its "flow" are necessary to attain occult enlightenment. For example, the yogic practice of *pranayama* attempts to use the breath to regulate the control of mystical life-energy "underneath" the breath, *prana*. The end goal is occultic enlightenment which frequently involves spirit contact and/or possession (see Question 43). Breath awareness methods have little to do with cardiovascular exercise. They are what the name implies—breath awareness or breath *meditation* (see Question 26).

## 12. What is (medical) channeling?

Medical channeling occurs when someone permits a spirit entity to possess him or her for New Age healing purposes. The spirits may possess the healer to perform psychic diagnosis or healing through them, or the spirits may use the vocal chords to speak through the person in order to give spiritual, medical, nutritional, and other teaching (see Question 18). Several forms of spirit communication by channeling exist, such as automatic writing and trance and inner voice dictation.

Increasingly, even medical doctors are turning to channelers for advice—or even becoming channelers themselves. For example, leading neurosurgeon C. Norman Shealy is the author of *Occult Medicine Can Save Your Life* and coauthor with Carolyn Myss of *The Creation of Health: Merging Traditional Medicine with Intuitive Diagnosis*. In his clinical practice he employs the psychic advice of spiritist Myss who channels an entity called "Genesis." Also, channeler Robert Leightman, M.D., an ordained Science of Mind minister, talks to spirits on a regular basis. With medium Carl Japikse, he is the coauthor of some 40 books of spiritistic revelation. His work as a psychic consultant to numerous medical doctors, psychiatrists, and psychologists has allegedly earned him a reputation as one of America's premier psychics.

Channeling claims to work through a variety of means. For example, by meditation, visualization, hypnosis, altered states of consciousness, and other methods, the spirits are able to enter, possess, and control a person much in the same way a puppeteer controls a puppet. New Age health therapists claim that by permitting spirits to possess and speak through them, mankind can attain a wealth of spiritual and other wisdom directly from spirits who have passed on or who are highly evolved. The spirits claim they can assist people's health concerns and direct them toward true individual and social enlightenment.

The major problem in channeling is that too much evidence exists that the spirits (who claim to be wise and loving entities sent from God to help people) are really lying spirits that the Bible identifies as demons. Channeling is part of what the Bible associates with the "spiritual forces of evil" (Ephesians 6:10-18) and is thus specifically forbidden (Deuteronomy 18:9-12). The hidden purpose of the spirits is to gain the trust of men so they can exert influence and control over them in order to bring about their eventual ruin.

Some of the potential dangers of channeling (as in all occultism) include spiritual deception, occult bondage, demon possession, mental breakdown, physical harm, and other consequences that we have documented in our *The Facts on Spirit Guides* and *The Facts on the Occult* (Harvest House).

## 13. What is chiropractic?

After medicine and dentistry, chiropractic is the largest health care system in the United States. Each year approximately 50,000 to 55,000 chiropractors treat 5 percent of the U.S. population. Chiropractic was invented by D.D. Palmer (1844-1913), a "magnetic" healer with an interest in spiritism. Chiropractic stresses the importance of the spine, believing that it is a vital organ of the body often neglected by contemporary medicine. Today, chiropractic theory and practice are frequently diverse and contradictory. Methods range from those which are responsible and scientific to those which are irresponsible and unscientific. Conflicting theory and practice means that almost any evaluation of chiropractic can be challenged as "unrepresentative." Nevertheless, the National Council Against Health Fraud's position paper on chiropractic, based on extensive research, claims that "most chiropractors do not share the view of health and disease held by health scientists worldwide." It supplies specific criteria which should be maintained by truly scientific practitioners of chiropractic.

It is important to realize that spinal manipulative therapy (SMT), used by chiropractors and many medical specialists such as physiatrists, is not necessarily the same as chiropractic. Manipulative therapy is safe, effective, and useful for treatment of back pain, headaches, and certain other musculoskeletal problems. Chiropractors are usually more skilled in this method than other practitioners because of their extensive training. But chiropractic as a whole may also involve more than manipulative therapy (incorporating additional treatments, some of which are New Age or scientifically questionable). Manipulative therapy itself may be overutilized by chiropractors or applied to conditions for which there is no known justification.

Chiropractic treatment involves physical adjustments to correct "subluxations" or misalignments of the spine. Spinal misalignments allegedly impinge or cause pressure upon spinal nerves, interfering with the flow of nerve impulses to the rest of the body, producing disease or susceptibility to disease. By correcting subluxations, proper performance of the nervous system is allegedly restored, thereby improving or maintaining health. This is why medical and other dictionaries characteristically define chiropractic as a system of treating disease based on spinal manipulation. Chiropractors also maintain that one of their principal concerns is the prevention of disease through the correction of subluxations.

Many chiropractors claim they can prevent or treat a significant number of illnesses and disorders that are unrelated to musculoskeletal problems. Chiropractic literature lists such conditions as high blood pressure, bronchial asthma, psychological problems, respiratory conditions, peptic ulcer, diabetes, heart trouble, etc. Practitioners believe that their clinical practice has produced results in improving or curing these conditions. They argue that such occasional clinical success means it is unfair to dismiss chiropractic's potential role in treating organic illness without further research.

Most medical texts note that the basic theory of chiropractic is not established and that chiropractic theory is not credible to the medical profession on the basis of current knowledge.

Writing in Scott Haldeman's (ed.) *Modern Developments in the Principles and Practice of Chiropractic* (1980, pp. 36,37) Walter I. Wardwell explains the dilemma:

> Chiropractors cannot have their cake and eat it too. To the extent that they reject the basic conceptions of medical science as fundamentally wrong, and propound chiropractic as a completely different philosophy and science capable of treating nearly the entire range of human ailments, they inevitably find great difficulty in convincing the mass of informed citizens that medicine's evaluation of chiropractic is wrong.

As an influential leader in the Christian Chiropractice Association told us, "No D.C. [Doctor of Chiropractic] wants to practice with medicine in any of its forms—pagan or scientific."

Chiropractors claim that what is already known about the nervous system and its regulation of the body makes the concept of the chiropractic subluxation at least possible. Simply because we can't prove the existence of subluxations or their effects is not the same as saying they cannot exist and have no influence on the body. In *Chiropractors: A Consumers' Guide* (p. 46), John Lagone argues: "No one knows enough about the working of the nervous system to say with certainty that chiropractic cannot do what it says it can do." Further, chiropractors maintain that medical doctors may "not understand the essential character of a subluxation" or may fail to note distinctions between *structural* defects which do not appear on X-ray and *functional* defects which will only become evident when a joint is examined through a range of motions.

Chiropractors also maintain that the results they obtain in their clinical practice indicate scientific research will eventually validate chiropractic theory.

Of course, if subluxations really help cause disease and chiropractors can remove them, thus helping cure disease, medical doctors and patients alike would be ecstatic. But even an article in the chiropractic journal *Journal of Manipulative and Physiological Therapeutics* (January 1991, p. 48) commented, "Perhaps even more harmful to the profession is the absence of its own body of scientific research confirming and explaining the precise pathogenic nature of the subluxation and the health-promoting qualities of its elimination."

Mark Bricklin, executive editor of *Prevention* magazine writes in *The Practical Encyclopedia of Natural Healing* (New York: Penguin, 1983-1990, p. 111): "Skeptics point out that there is no proof, no clinical evidence suggesting that if the spinal column is 'like that of a newborn's'—clear of obstruction—there will be no disease. Or that chiropractic manipulations can be expected to speed relief of anything more than aches and pains of the musculoskeletal system."

Critics wonder why of all the medical specialists in the world, only chiropractors are found to accept subluxations. As Hank Pizer, a noted medical writer observes in his *Guide to the New Medicine: What Works, What Doesn't* (New York: William Morrow, 1982, p. 83), "The 'subluxation' that chiropractors refer to appears to be largely a theoretical construct accepted primarily by chiropractors."

Science writer and chiropractic advocate John Lagone observes (p. 27) that "all chiropractors agree that the subluxation plays a role in disease and disorder. But their opinions differ as to what part of the body subluxation is found in, over how important it is to specific diseases and malfunctions, and over what constitutes proper treatment."

Dr. William T. Jarvis is professor of prevention medicine at Loma Linda University and president of the National Council Against Health Fraud. He was awarded his Ph.D. for research on chiropractic. He writes as a critic of chiropractic and seeks to spur reform within the industry. In *Ministry* (May 1990, p. 26) he observes that chiropractors have never defined a subluxation in measurable terms, nor proven that it exists. He notes that in spite of the ability of neurophysiologists to measure nerve impulses, chiropractors have never shown that impinging a spinal nerve alters an impulse beyond the zone of impingement or that disrupting a nerve impulse can produce disease. He cites the important anatomical research of Yale University anatomist Edmund Crelin as having demonstrated that subluxations cannot function in the manner chiropractic claims. He also maintains that many studies have been conducted in which two or more chiropractors were unable to find the same subluxations either on the same X-ray or in the same patients, indicating that chiropractors can easily disagree over what specific conditions require treatment.

If subluxations exist and if there really is a chance that correcting them can cure disease, this would be wonderful. But this needs to be demonstrated by standard research. Relying upon the claims or experience of empirical medicine leaves one uncertain that the noted effects aren't attributable to other causes.

Nevertheless, appropriate physical manipulation employed by chiropractors can be both safe and beneficial. General massage for headaches and rational conservative spinal manipulation therapy for some backaches and other neuromusculoskeletal disorders is medically justifiable. This is why most chiropractors apparently spend most of their time in treating neuromusculoskeletal symptoms. The *British Medical Journal* (June 2, 1990) reports that chiropractic "was more effective" for certain types of severe back pain than standard hospital outpatient management. The 1991 *Rand Report* concluded the following (p. V):

> The literature on the efficacy of spinal manipulaton is of uneven quality.... Given that caveat, support is consistent for the use of spinal manipulation as a treatment for patients with acute low-back pain and an absence of other signs or symptoms of lower limb nerve-root involvement. Support is less clear for the other indications, with the evidence for some insufficient (acute and subacute low-back pain with sciatica, acute and subacute low-back pain with

minor lower limb neurologic findings, most types of chronic back pain), while the evidence for others is conflicting (acute low-back pain with sciatica and minor lower limb neurological findings, subacute low-back pain without sciatica, and chronic low-back pain without sciatica).

Chiropractic, like dentistry, is a limited specialty that should not replace standard medical care. Responsible chiropractors are good physical therapists, not primary care physicians.

Although chiropractic itself is not New Age, unfortunately many chiropractors employ many of the holistic health treatments cited in this booklet. Some commentators believe chiropractic may play a key role in the advancement of holistic health in this country. Also, early chiropractic theory (incorporating a belief in a divine life-force called "Innate") may open the door to occultic practices or beliefs among chiropractors who hold to this or similar views.

In addition, a number of New Age therapies have been developed by chiropractors—such as iridology, developed by Bernard Jensen; applied kinesiology, developed by George Goodhart; Touch for Health, developed by John Thie; and naprapathy, developed by Oakley G. Smith. Unfortunately, chiropractic almost single-handedly began the fallacious practice of "muscle testing" in this country (see Question 27). We have also encountered a number of people who have become actual teachers of New Age therapies principally because their personal chiropractor used a particular New Age treatment on them, sparking their interest. Reflexology, iridology, homeopathy, and polarity therapy are examples.

The acceptance of undemonstrated theories or New Age methods that are found in modern chiropractic means that practitioners of chiropractic should be carefully evaluated before a patient begins treatment. The significant Christian influence within chiropractic *should* be at the forefront of reform within the industry.

## 14. What is chromotherapy/color therapy?

Color therapy involves the alleged psychic use and perception of color to diagnose and treat physical illness and/or emotional problems. For example, color therapists claim they can accurately diagnose the condition of the body by psychically "seeing" and evaluating the condition of the "aura," an alleged psychic sheath surrounding living things, or the *chakras*, alleged psychic centers within the body. They claim that prescribing appropriate "color treatments" or "energy channeling" will correct color/vibration deficiencies in the aura and/or *chakras*, helping to heal the body.

The field of chromotherapy is replete with subjective practices and conflicting beliefs, making objective diagnosis and treatment impossible. Chromotherapy is almost always either an occultic practice and/or fraud. Examples of occultic potential found in chromotherapy treatments include psychic development, energy channeling, occultic meditation, and development of altered states of consciousness.

Complications arising from color therapy could include misdiagnosis of a serious illness or susceptibility to occultic influences. Color therapy should be distinguished from the legitimate scientific study of color and its effects upon animals and humans.

### 15. What is crystal healing/crystal work?

Crystal healing, currently one of the most popular New Age practices, is the use of a supposed "power" inherent within crystals for healing, developing psychic abilities, spirit contact, and other New Age goals. Crystals supposedly contain the ability to focus and direct psychic energies for healing and other occult pursuits.

Crystal work is a form of animism in which inanimate objects are held to possess spiritual powers that may be contacted, utilized, or directed. But in animism any supernatural power contacted originates from the spirit world. Thus, crystals *per se* have no magical powers and only become an implement behind which spirits may work. When pressed, most crystal healers we have talked with concede that the power behind crystals is spiritistic.

Many similar objects are also believed to possess magical properties (amulets, magical stones, or gems), but one fact discounts this belief: Psychic abilities and powers remain once the implement is dispensed with. In other words, these objects are only contact material—a disguise through which spirits work to gain influence over people's lives.

All divinatory methods utilize some principle object that becomes the focus and/or vehicle through which spirits work to serve the client and produce the needed answer to questions, character analysis, future prognostication, supernatural power, etc. Common forms of divination and the objects they use include astrology (the horoscope chart); tarot (a deck of cards with symbols); I Ching (sticks, printed hexagrams); runes (dice); Ouija board (an alphabet plan-chette); radionics/psychometry (the divining rod, pendulum, "black box," etc.); palmistry (the hand); crystal-gazing (the crystal ball or crystal rock); metoscopy/physiognomy/phre-nology (the forehead, face, skull); geomancy (combinations of dots or points); water dowsing (the forked stick or other object).

Is it logical to expect that mere pieces of paper bearing symbols (horoscopes), simple forked sticks, cards, hands, dice, letters of the alphabet, rocks, facial lines, or dots could ever supply supernatural power or miraculous information about a person or their future? Even the practitioners of these arts refer to "supernatural influences"—to "gods" and spirits who operate through these methods.

The potential problems arising from crystal healing include those of New Age Medicine in general: misdiagnosis, mistreatment, and occultic influence.

## 16. What is dowsing, water dowsing?

Dowsing is a psychic practice employing divinatory implements (e.g., rod and pendulum, forked sticks) and methods in order to search out desired information. For example, dowsing is used to discover the nature or location of disease and determine the proper treatment. It is also used to locate water or minerals, lost objects, missing persons, buried treasure, etc. Water dowsing claims to work through a supposedly natural sensitivity to geomagnetic phenomena, "water radiations," or by some allegedly unconscious "motor ability" operating in an unknown manner.

But dowsing is not the human ability that many people assume it is. Rather, it is a spiritistic power (see Question 33). Learning to dowse often involves the cultivation of mild to moderate altered states of consciousness, the development of psychic powers, and even spirit contact. As documented in dowsing literature itself or in Ben Hester's *Dowsing: An Exposé of Hidden Occult Forces* (self-published: available from 4883 Hedrick Ave., Arlington, CA 92505), many leading dowsers freely confess that dowsing is a supernatural ability, and some also confess to having spirit guides.

Biblically, dowsing is rejected both by description (Hosea 4:12) and by nature (as divination, Deuteronomy 18:9-12).

Some of the potential dangers of dowsing include health risks through improper diagnosis or treatment, occultic influences, and financial loss or other deception through dowsing failures.

## 17. What is dream work?

Dreams fascinate millions of people, including a large number of researchers. Dream work involves the exploration of and/or interaction with dreams as an adjunct to physical healing, for psychological insight in psychotherapy, for spiritual insight in "Christian" dream work, and/or the manipulation of dreams for occultic revelations or spiritual growth in New Age practices.

Dream work practices, which extend into antiquity, claim that our dreams can powerfully reflect and/or influence physical, psychological, and spiritual realities. In physical healing, dreams may allegedly be used to reveal hindrances and provide assistance to the healing process. In psychotherapy, exploring dreams may allegedly open doors to the unconscious mind to reveal and help resolve hidden emotional conflicts or other problems. In Christian dream work, dreams are seen as signs or even personal messages or revelations from God; therefore, for some, exploring dreams is equivalent to studying "God's Word." In New Age practices dreams can be explored and even manipulated, as in lucid dream work. In lucid dream work, dreams are employed for various reasons, including occultic revelation, spirit contact, psychic development, astral travel, and to induce altered states of consciousness.

Considerable research has been done on the nature, purpose and meaning of dreams; however, much still remains tentative.

The major problems with dream work are as follows: (1) the value of dream work to physical healing is unsubstantiated; (2) dream work interpretation in psychotherapy and other therapies is often subjective and contradictory; (3) in psychotherapeutic and "Christian" dream work, and in New Age occultic manipulation of dreams, the practice may have unexpected or unforeseen consequences. For example, some researchers have speculated that dream work may inhibit the normal process of forgetting damaging experiences; (4) many of the dream-work books and manuals we consulted promoted spirit contact under the guise of dialoguing with "dream characters." Dream work can also be used for other occult purposes, explaining why spirit guides frequently encourage the practice (e.g., the spiritistic revelations found in such books as *Edgar Cayce on Dreams* and Jane Roberts' *Seth: Dreams and Projection of Consciousness*).

Perhaps it is best that normal dreams are not given a spiritual or other significance they do not possess. Divinely inspired dreams such as those found in the Bible are (1) relatively rare, (2) given by God to accomplish His will, (3) unable to be induced or manipulated by man, and (4) clear in purpose and meaning. God's use of dreams in the Bible stands in contrast to their common use in psychotherapy, Christian dream work, and occultic dream manipulation where their value and meaning are unestablished.

## 18. What are the Edgar Cayce methods of healing?

Edgar Cayce's books have sold multiple millions of copies, all of them stressing the importance of health. The Edgar Cayce methods of healing involve a health program and philosophy based on the spiritistic revelations (called "Readings") of medium Edgar Cayce (1877-1944). By following the health suggestions given in these occult readings, it is claimed that one will maintain optimum health. The health suggestions combine natural therapies, such as castor oil packs, with "proper" mental attitudes (attitudinal healing, see Question 5) and "proper" spiritual (occult) "attunement."

While Edgar Cayce channeled the information concerning healing, specific programs based on it have been developed in conjunction with the official Cayce organization, the Association for Research and Enlightenment (ARE) in Virginia Beach, Virginia. A significant number of medical doctors have been converted to Cayce's methods, which are also promoted by various Cayce clinics, referral programs, and dozens of ARE symposia on New Age medicine offered over the years.

Based on known scientific data, most if not all of Cayce's methods have been discredited. If they work, they work for reasons unrelated to the given theories. For example, the treatments work far better for those who have adopted Cayce's occultic worldview, suggesting psychological and occultic components to healing. Even leaders in the Cayce methods of health such as Dr. Harold J. Reilly have admitted that the methods usually work only for those who believe in Cayce's occultic philosophy.

The major problem with this approach is that Cayce's "Readings" are not based upon the findings of scientific medicine. Rather, they are integrated with reincarnation philosophy, healing by "vibrational" correspondences,* and other New Age occultic ideas. Because the "Readings" teach

---

* alleged psychic connections between the body and the universe, or the body and a patient's "medicine"

that "health" is promoted by a "proper" mental and/or spiritual attitude, people who use Cayce's revelations as part of a health program often end up with an occultic worldview.

Spiritistic revelations on any subject should not be trusted, because any truth given is always mixed with serious spiritual or other error. The dangers of the Cayce methods involve conversion to occultism and the fact that the treatments suggested by the "Readings" may be ineffective, false, or dangerous.

## 19. What is herbal medicine (botanotherapy, phytotherapy, aromatherapy, vegotherapy)?

Herbal medicine is the use of herbs and other plant products to allegedly help cure a wide variety of physical ailments, or the use of "spiritually potentized" herbs and plants for physical or psychic healing and/or other occult pursuits—as in the Bach Flower Remedies, Vita Florum, aromatherapy, and similar practices. Particular herbs, plants, or flowers are believed to possess physical or spiritual healing properties. Roots, leaves, stems, plants, seeds, etc., are prepared in various ways, sometimes through psychic methods, and either consumed orally as medicine or used on the skin as ointment.

Some herbs and plants do contain medicinal properties and in extracted or synthetic forms are used in modern health care and medical treatment. The scientific discipline known as pharmacognosy is a legitimate and important field, but extensive scientific research is required to separate the wheat from the chaff. Unfortunately, New Age herbalism largely ignores scientific concerns and pursues its own methods and interests.

For example, New Age herbal medicine may incorporate practices such as developing altered states of consciousness and spirit contact through use of hallucinogenic plants (as in many forms of shamanism) or practicing psychic healing through regulating a supposed occult power latent within plants and herbs.

New Age herbal medicine is largely, if not exclusively, a combination of questionable commercialism and wishful thinking based on ignorance (cf. V.E. Tyler, *The Honest Herbal*). Many commonly sold herbal remedies, even some herbal teas, are potentially harmful by themselves or through allergic reactions or synergism. Some remedies contain plant products that are carcinogenic and others are mislabeled or found to be contaminated with insect parts. Further, using ineffective or dangerous treatments may delay or otherwise acerbate serious illness, and one may also encounter other occult influences through New Age herbalism.

## 20. What is homeopathy?

Homeopathy is the system of diagnosis and treatment developed by medical rebel and mystic Samuel Hahnemann (1755-1843). It is based on the principle of "like cures like"— that the same substance causing symptoms in a healthy person will cure those symptoms in a sick person. In Europe, homeopathy is increasingly accepted by the medical profession and in America, several thousand homeopaths treat hundreds of thousands of satisfied customers.

Homeopathy claims to work by correcting an imbalance or problem in the body's "vital force" or life-energy that is currently or will later be manifested as disease. By an almost ritual process of diluting and shaking, homeopathic substances (alleged medications) supposedly become powerful energy medicines which in turn either stimulate the immune system or correct problems in the supposed "vital force" of the body, thereby curing the illness.

There are three different kinds of practicing homeopaths: (1) the traditional homeopath who largely follows the unscientific and potentially occultic theories of Samuel Hahnemann; (2) the scientifically and/or parapsychologically oriented homeopath who attempts to bring homeopathy into the twentieth century, including, however, the highly suspect practice of almost infinitely diluting its "medications"; and (3) the "demythologized" homeopath who thinks homeopathic medicines may work through unknown principles, but questions that homeopathic medicines can be effective in dilution so high that literally not one molecule of the original "medicine" remains.

Despite many claims and alleged parallels to modern medical practices and phenomena, homeopathy is not a legitimate medical practice. Homeopathic diagnosis is subjective and ineffective; most homeopathic "medicines" are so dilute they cannot possibly exert a physical effect. The claim that they work upon the "vital force" or "astral body" is unsubstantiated and can open doors to occult practices.

Homeopaths refer to some 20 or more studies that they claim confirm the value of homeopathy, yet ignore innumerable studies which disprove homeopathic "laws." Of course, with literally thousands of plant, mineral, and animal homeopathic substances being widely tested, marketed, and consumed (everything from deadly nightshade, snake venom, arsenic, and gunpowder to sand, cockroach, and lobster) it is at least possible, at low dilutions, that a few might be found to have medicinal value (see Question 19). But each substance would require stringent testing to prove its effectiveness. Further, this would not prove homeopathy true. It would only prove that the actual preexisting medicinal properties of certain substances (not their "vital force") were being employed and that these were having a *physical* effect, not an occult one.

Examples of the occult potential of homeopathic diagnosis and treatment include homeopaths who employ: psychic diagnosis and healing; spiritism; astrology and other occult philosophies; and the use of pendulums, radionic instruments, and other occult devices.

## 21. What are hypnosis and hypnotic regression?

Hypnosis is a deliberately induced condition of heightened suggestibility and trance, producing a highly flexible state of consciousness capable of dramatic manipulation. It is employed by thousands of medical professionals and psychotherapists.

The practice can be traced to antiquity and is frequently associated with the occult. The hypnotist and psychic Anton Mesmer (from whom we derive the term "mesmerism") is often considered the modern father of hypnosis.

The exact processes by which hypnosis works are unknown. Scientific research has been conducted supplying much information on the level of hypnotic trance and susceptibility to it; nevertheless, what hypnosis is and how it works are still widely debated. Widespread and frequently exaggerated claims are made for its application to medicine, psychotherapy, education, and many other fields. Some self-help promoters make sensational claims that hypnosis can be used to treat or cure an endless variety of physical ailments and personal problems—from allergies, obesity, and cancer to low self-esteem, smoking, and guilt. They allege that its potential application to personal growth, human potentialism, and self-transformation is nearly endless.

We readily agree that hypnosis is a unique altered state of consciousness that can be used for a wide variety of occult pursuits—including psychic development, spirit contact, astral travel, automatic writing, past-life (reincarnation) regression and/or therapy, and many others. But as we have documented in *The Facts on the Occult* and *The Facts on Hinduism in America* (Harvest House), such practices are dangerous.

Other problems also present themselves with the use of hypnosis, not the least of which is the release of one's mind to the suggestions and control of another person, as well as possible uncertainties as to the nature and long-term implications of the hypnotic state. It is also at least possible that hypnosis may be related to the biblically forbidden practice of "charming" and/or "enchanting." If so, the practice would be prohibited in that the Christian is to be filled with the Holy Spirit; he is not to permit his mind to be controlled by another person, in particular an unbeliever, or to permit the possibility of influence by spirit entities, as in certain occultic applications of hypnosis.

Other risks of hypnosis include the possibility of unintended and unexpected occultic influences or other problems arising from the trance state, and abuse by the hypnotist.

In addition, literally scores of New Age and some conventional psychotherapists employ what is called "past-life therapy." Over a dozen texts by licensed psychologists have been written on this topic. Past-life therapy employs hypnosis to place the individual into a trance state for a specific purpose. That purpose is to send the person "back" into his or her supposed former life or lives in order to resolve hidden emotional or spiritual conflicts that are allegedly affecting his or her physical, emotional, or spiritual health at the present. But the results of such therapy are typically to support occultic New Age philosophy and goals.

Our own extensive research into reincarnation phenomena leads us to conclude that these and other reincarnation experiences are the result of one or more factors: (1) the suggestions of the therapist, (2) the inventions or delusions of the patient, or (3) the spiritistic manipulation of the mind.

Hypnosis can easily induce a state of trance conducive to spiritistic manipulation. Because reincarnation philosophy is so antibiblical in its implications and the entire purpose of past-life regression is to encounter alleged previous lives, spiritistic input is hardly out of the question. Even some leading secular researchers such as Dr. Ian Stevenson of the University of Virginia have confessed that possession by an evil spirit is one of the possible explanations for reincarnation phenomena (*Twenty Cases Suggestive of Reincarnation*, 1978, pp. 374 ff.).

People who have these "past-life" experiences can be profoundly affected by them, and they not infrequently lead to occult involvement. They may produce dramatic life and worldview changes. For example, the individual who comes to believe in reincarnation through past-life regression is convinced that when he dies, he will not encounter divine judgment as the Bible teaches, but simply another life. Thus, one who believes in reincarnation cannot logically accept his or her need to believe in Christ as savior from sin. If he will atone for his own sins over many lifetimes through *karma* and achieve his own perfection, why does he need a savior?

But the Bible rejects all philosophies of reincarnation. If Christ paid for all sin upon the cross, one sacrifice for all time (Hebrews 9:26-28; 10:14), what sin remains for us to individually atone for over many lifetimes? The atonement of Christ disproves the karmic theory of a gradual remission of sin and self-perfection just as the biblical doctrine of individual resurrection disproves the idea that we progress through many lifetimes in different bodies.

Unfortunately, past-life therapy has often become a form of occultic practice leading patients to adopt an occultic worldview and to seek out such activities as developing altered states of consciousness, psychic powers, and spirit contact. Because of the subtlety of the spiritual implications involved, past-life therapy is no less profound in its destructive potential than similar areas where spiritual warfare is unsuspected but nonetheless pervasive. For example, near-death experiences and the phenomenon of UFO "close encounter" episodes both frequently induce occultic initiations and transformation in a subject.

## 22. What is (New Age) intuition?

New Age intuition is a euphemism for a wide variety of New Age psychic and occultic powers. New Age intuition is frequently employed with occultic healing, telepathy, clairvoyance, psychic diagnosis, and spiritism. "Intuition" is developed in the same manner as psychic abilities (e.g., training programs involving meditation, concentration, altered states of consciousness, etc.). Once developed, a person seeks out his intuitive abilities and relies on their guidance and instruction for whatever healing or other tasks are at hand.

The basic problem with New Age intuition is its unjustified parapsychological premise: the normalization of psychic powers as "intuitive abilities" latent to the human race. This masks their true reality as supernatural abilities originating in conjunction with the spirit world.* Occult abilities and spiritistic powers are thus psychologically

---

* See our *The Facts on the Occult* (Harvest House, 1990).

internalized as part of latent "human potential"; intuition *per se*, a normal human process, becomes a cover for occultism, while spiritual warfare goes on behind the scenes. Thus, distinguishing one's perception of normal human intuition from psychic powers becomes difficult or impossible. In fact, it is frightening to realize that many spiritists confess that they are unable to distinguish their own spirit guide's influence upon their minds from normal human inspiration or creativity. This means that those people who open themselves to the influence of the spirit world can be manipulated by spirits imperceptibly.

Biblically, occultic practices are forbidden, no matter what they are called (Deuteronomy 18:9-12). The dangers of New Age intuition include fostering occult development under the guise of enhancing normal human intuition, along with the normal physical, mental, and spiritual hazards associated with occult practice.

## 23. What is iridology?

Iridology is the study of the iris of the human eye to allegedly diagnose present and even future illness and disease. Ignatz von Peczely (1822-1911) is considered the modern developer; however, similar practices can be seen in ancient Chinese methods related to astrology. Occultist Bernard Jensen is considered the leading U.S. authority.

Iridologists claim that the eyes can mirror the health condition of the body because the iris allegedly displays in detail the status of every organ system. Supposedly, the iris's connection with the central nervous system permits detailed information to be sent from the rest of the body back to the iris. Further, according to iridology theory, each iris reveals what is happening on its own side of the body, an anatomical impossibility. (Incoming nerve impulses from one side of the body almost always cross to the opposite side on their way to the brain.)

Iridology has been discredited in numerous scientific studies and is, therefore, a form of health fraud. Some of these studies are reported in the *Journal of the American Medical Association* (September 28, 1979), *Australian Journal of Optometry* (July 1982), and *Journal of the American Optometric Association* (October 1984). Despite its lack of credibility, iridology is increasingly accepted, even when used as or in conjunction with psychic diagnosis and healing.

The problems associated in using iridology include the progression of a serious illness that iridology fails to uncover, personal anxiety and loss of finances from misdiagnosis that a serious illness exists, and spiritual problems from occultic influences in occult forms.

## 24. What is Kirlian photography?

Kirlian photography is a controversial method of photography developed by Russian electrical technician Semyon Kirlian. It allegedly reveals a corona or "aura" around living things. Occultists frequently claim this photography supplies evidence of man's inner psychic nature related to his alleged "astral body," "higher self," or occult aura. Psychics also claim to see auras around people, which are said to interpret their physical, emotional, or spiritual condition. Allegedly, Kirlian photography reveals this aura that psychics claim to see. Kirlian photography is also said to offer evidence of the healing abilities of psychics and spiritists insofar as it reveals the existence of the "astral body," "higher self," or other psychic components to man variously related to the healing process that occultists claim to employ.

But the meaning and value of Kirlian photography are not known and New Age occultic interpretations are doubtful at best. Occult interpretations of this phenomena frequently associate it with mystical occult energies connected with spiritism which are then wrongly interpreted as divine, natural, or neutral energies (see Question 31).

No one denies there are weak electrical phenomena within the body or that living entities have what could be interpreted as "energy" fields. For example, the electroencephalograph can detect electrodynamic phenomena in the brain, and other instruments can detect heat energy radiating from our bodies. But to say that these supply any evidence for the occultic concept of the "aura" or the occultic energy called *prana, chi, ki,* etc., would be wrong. New Agers may speak of the thermal or electrical activity of the body as "bioenergy," but it should not in any way be confused with the "aura," or the *prana, mana, ki, chi,* etc., of New Age medicine. Comparing the scientific descriptions of known bodily phenomena to the occultic descriptions of the aura reveals that both the "fields" and "energies" are vastly different.

Exactly what the Kirlian photography reveals is still uncertain. Kirlian photography may have experimental uses, but not for New Age believers. Its phenomena are explainable by recourse to more mundane things such as human sweat or the photographing process itself.

As noted, New Age interpretations of Kirlian phenomena are cited as evidence of a human aura that many psychics claim to see. But first, not every psychic claims to be able to see auras. One wonders why if everyone supposedly has an aura that can be psychically perceived. Second, if auras are universal to man and internally generated by the human body or spirit, they should be able to be seen in the dark. But not all psychics can see them in the dark.

Third, Kirlian photography reveals auras around everything—inanimate objects such as coins and desks included—not just people, leaves, or other living things. This also suggests that the Kirlian phenomenon is related to the photographic process. Biblically, we know that inanimate objects do not contain a spiritual essence. Thus, whatever Kirlian photography reveals, it does not appear to be something spiritual. If it reveals the same aura around dead objects that cannot have a spirit or spiritual life, why should we conclude that the aura it reveals around living objects is anything spiritual? Fourth, whatever psychics are seeing does not appear to be genuine psychic perception of the human spirit or some universal, mystical energy field because the reports psychics give are too dissimilar and contradictory.

Finally, any known bodily energy or electricity is much too weak to become a healing power or the source of psychic abilities which occultists claim. And if everyone has an inner core of mystical divine power, then everyone should be able to develop psychic powers. But, in fact, the only ones who do so are occultists who have spirit guides.

## 25. What are the martial arts (aikido, tai chi chuan, tae kwon do, karate, judo, kenpo, ninjutsu, etc.)?

The martial arts are systems of physical discipline stressing the control of mind and body for self-defense, health, and often, spiritual "enlightenment." Different methods have different founders and emphases. The martial arts claim to work by unifying the mind/spirit and body through meditation, physical discipline, and other procedures. This allegedly helps to 1) regulate the flow of mystical energy throughout the body (ki in Japanese; chi in Chinese) and 2) enable one to attain a state of mind-body oneness. Both elements are deemed important to effective performance of self-defense techniques and/or "enlightenment."

The major problem with the martial arts is that people who attend a martial arts program only for physical purposes may easily be converted to the underlying philosophy of the particular system being practiced. Because most methods incorporate Eastern teachings and techniques, the martial arts constitute an excellent opportunity for conversion to Taoism, Buddhism, and other East Asian religions. Further, some martial arts programs involve occult meditation, development of psychic powers, and even spirit contact (e.g., *Somatics*, Vol. 4, No. 3, pp. 48-49).

Because the martial arts or their precursors were originally developed in Greece and only later incorporated the occultism of the East, in theory, the martial arts can be a neutral technique of profound physical development. This is not to say that neutral forms of the martial arts can necessarily be developed in every method; some may be inextricably bound to Eastern theory and practice. Any program having Eastern or occultic beliefs or methods should be avoided.

Further, we should not underestimate the delicate issue when a person is converted from martial arts practice to Christian faith. Such a person may find it essential to forsake all association with his former ways as a requirement to spiritual growth. Also, the modern orientation toward offensive procedures may make the issue of Christian participation problematic. The martial arts are extremely demanding physically. Thus, besides the possibility of occultic influence in Eastern forms, some serious physical hazards (such as head injury) may present themselves by the very nature of martial arts practice. An article in the *Taekwondo Times* (January 1987, p. 84), "Neurological Disorders in the Martial Arts," by Dr. Michael Trulson, cautions that "head injuries are the most commonly ignored serious injuries in the martial arts. Often they are not taken seriously and fatalities occur that could easily have been prevented."

## 26. What is (New Age) meditation?

New Age (Eastern-occultic) meditation is practiced by millions of people. It involves the control and regulation of the mind for various physical and spiritual (occult) purposes. Meditation promoters claim the practice has numerous health benefits, but even if true, the potential spiritual and even physical hazards outweigh them. Meditation claims to work by "stilling" or otherwise influencing the mind. The meditator is allegedly able to perceive true reality, his own true nature, and to achieve true spiritual enlightenment. The majority of forms of meditation practiced today are occultic. In his *The Varieties of Meditative Experience* (p. 117), meditation authority Dr. Daniel

Goleman observes: "Virtually every system of meditation recognizes the awakened state as the ultimate goal of meditation. . . . Each path labels this end state differently. But no matter how diverse the names, these paths all propose the same basic formula in an alchemy [occultic transformation] of the self."

Apart from a "relaxation response," scientific studies have confirmed other physical and psychological influences of meditation, but their meaning and value are widely interpreted.

New Age meditation characteristically uses the mind in an abnormal manner to radically restructure a person's perceptions toward supporting occultic philosophy and goals. Regressive or spiritistically induced states of consciousness are wrongly interpreted as "higher" or "divine" states of consciousness. For example, in many forms of meditation practice, spirit possession itself is actually interpreted as a form of spiritual enlightenment; further, meditation-developed psychic powers are falsely interpreted as evidence of a latent divine nature. Unfortunately, meditators often do not realize the possible long-term results or consequences of these practices. For example, the dangerous and growing phenomenon of *kundalini* arousal (see Question 43) characteristically incorporates periods of severe mental disruption and demonization.

The underlying philosophy, stated purpose, physical method, and spiritual context of meditation determine its outcome. Responsible biblical meditation is a spiritually healthy practice; but again, most meditation practiced today involves occultic methods which may bring harmful consequences. Among them are spiritistic influence and even demon possession, and various forms of physical, psychological, and spiritual damage which are increasingly reported in the literature.

## 27. What is muscle testing (applied kinesiology, Touch for Health, behavioral kinesiology)?

"Muscle testing" is one of the fastest growing alternative health care techniques in the United States. Muscle testing programs vary but are frequently a combination of chiropractic and Chinese acupuncture theory plus muscle testing itself. First, these programs involve physical diagnosis by testing the supposed strength or weakness of muscles which are believed to be related to organ systems. Weak muscles allegedly reflect "energy" depletion in corresponding organs, producing susceptibility to disease. In the "challenge technique" an agent suspected of causing physical

harm (anything from white sugar and other foods to pre-
scription medicine) is held in the mouth or hand. Then, the
therapist "proves" its weakening effect upon the body by
alleged display of the patient's weakened muscle resis-
tance. Other methods (e.g., "therapy localization") use
mere touch to diagnose or heal.

Second, these programs may employ treatment or healing by alleged regulation of "cosmic" energies, acupressure,
meridian tracing, chiropractic, and other methods. Muscle
testing often claims to manipulate alleged body energies to
produce and maintain healing. By supposedly unblocking
congested energy along meridian pathways and/or infusing
energy into deficient systems or bodily areas, practitioners
believe that physical health can be improved.

Muscle testing frequently rejects the known facts of
human anatomy and claims to treat bodily energies whose
existence has never been proven. Further, its manipulation
of such invisible energies can become an occultic practice,
e.g., a form of psychic or absent (at a distance) healing.
Muscle testers may also employ occult devices such as pendulums, dowsing instruments, and other radionic devices
(see Questions 15,16). Because it is an unsubstantiated
practice that is characteristically based on Taoist philosophy or other Eastern metaphysics and is potentially occultic, it should be avoided. Christian practitioners claim
that they avoid the occult when they are manipulating
energy, but how can they be sure they are (1) doing anything at all, or (2) actually avoiding the occult?

Modern muscle testing must be distinguished from the
*scientific* discipline of kinesiology. Formal kinesiology is
the study of the principles of mechanics and anatomy in
relation to human movement, or the science of human muscular movements. It is frequently used in physical education and therapy. While muscle testing may or may not
employ some of the methods and theories of formal kinesiology, scientific kinesiology never employs the methods of
New Age muscle testing. The two disciplines are based on
different approaches to physiology and health.

## 28. What is naturopathy?

Naturopathy is an approach to health and disease which
assumes that natural methods of treatment are preferable
to synthetic treatments such as drugs and surgery. Naturopathy is based on the idea that illness is due to an accumu-
lation of toxins or waste products in the body. Physical
symptoms are the body's attempt to rid itself of these toxins.

The basic problem with naturopathy is that its methods are characteristically ineffective when confronting serious illness, and its bias against modern medicine only compounds the problem. Further, the definition of "natural" is frequently subjective; "natural" treatment may include the methods of occultic medicine. Here, naturopathy employs a wide range of New Age treatments having occultic potential such as radionics, homeopathy, meditation, and yoga. Thus, naturopathy may inhibit correct diagnosis of a problem, permitting a curable illness to assume serious or incurable proportions; it may also offer ineffective treatments and involve clients in occultic methods. Nevertheless, with theoretical revision and practical safeguards, naturopathy could function as a commendable model for preventive health care and treatment of minor ailments. However, Christian enthusiasts should exercise caution; naturopathy as a whole is part of New Age medicine.

## 29. What is osteopathy?

Today, osteopathic physicians hold traditional medical degrees and, therefore, generally employ scientific medicine. While in practice, most osteopaths may be little different from conventional physicians, some seek to maintain the distinctives of their profession. Classical osteopathy is the practice of physical manipulation designed to help restore the body's health. Developed by Andrew Taylor Still (1828-1917), an eccentric country doctor interested in metaphysics, osteopathy sees body structure and function as interdependent; thus, abnormal structure may affect the functions of the physical body. If the physician can restore proper structure, health should improve and/or be maintained.

Certain osteopathic concepts present problems. For example, the osteopathic lesion (in nature and importance similar to the chiropractic subluxation) is not scientifically demonstrated. Further, some theories and approaches of traditional or in some cases modern osteopaths, such as "cranial osteopathy," are rejected by medical science. Further, conventional medicine does not place the degree of importance upon the musculoskeletal system or accept the claims of some osteopaths concerning its relation to organ function.

On the other hand, some osteopathic research, as with chiropractic research, may prove valuable because it is investigating new areas unique to these disciplines. As a whole, osteopathy appears to present legitimate but occasionally marginal or suspect medical practice. One also finds infrequent New Age Edgar Cayce associations related to some early theories and modern practices of osteopathy.

## 30. What is polarity therapy?

Polarity therapy is the practice of channeling energy from the healer into the client to allegedly restore or balance the body's repository of mystical energy (*chi, prana*) believed to flow between positive and negative "poles" in the body. Founded by occultist Randolph Stone, polarity therapy claims that "sore" spots are first located to determine where *chi* blockage exists; the Polarity Zone Chart then determines the organ or part of the body to which the "sore spot" responds. By channeling psychic energy through the therapist's hands, the flow of *chi* is restored to corresponding body organs. These practices, plus the addition of other methods (e.g., acupressure, bioenergetics, yoga, self-hypnosis, energy astrology) and practices (e.g., diet, special exercises, mental affirmations), are believed to maintain physical and spiritual health.

The practices of polarity therapy have never been established to work on the basis of their stated principles. Further, as in therapeutic touch, most people have wrongly concluded that this is not an occultic method because of its innocent appearance. Yet polarity therapy is a form of psychic healing involving energy channeling and, potentially, spiritism. Along with other forms of psychic healing, the potential dangers include misdiagnosis, mistreatment, and occultic influences.

## 31. What are psychic anatomies (astral bodies, meridians, auras, chakras, nadis)?

Psychic anatomies are alleged invisible, nonphysical, inner "structures" frequently associated with Eastern/occult religions, related to mystical energy, and often employed in New Age diagnosis and healing. These structures were apparently first noted psychically by occultists having spirit guides in various pagan religious traditions. New Age healers who utilize these structures claim that they help reveal physical, mental, and sometimes spiritual illness even before it manifests on the physical or mental level.

Use of these "anatomies" is characteristically dependent upon altered states of consciousness, psychic development, and/or the spirit contact necessary to "see" and "influence" them.

Theoretically, such inner structures could exist, although this is doubtful because those who claim to psychically see them offer contradictory reports as to their number, nature, and function. For example, the numbers of astral bodies range from 1-9; meridians from 72-2,000, *chakras* from 6-12, and *nadis* from 72,000-326,000. Further, their almost universal association with occultism and the need for occultic development to use them negates any claim to a neutral science of psychic anatomies. Thus, various contradictions in theory and practice belie the claim that these structures can be used in any objective manner in medical diagnosis and treatment.

## 32. What are psychic diagnosis, psychic healing, and psychic surgery?

These are ancient spiritistic methods of diagnosis and healing performed supernaturally in conjunction with spirit guides whose presence may or may not be evident to the healer or client. Practitioners claim that they diagnose, heal, or even perform "surgery" through altered states of consciousness, radionic devices, and/or spirit guides. Such spiritism is often masked under New Age, psychological, or parapsychological concepts such as the "higher self," "inner counselor," Jungian "archetypes," or latent psychic ability, etc. But whatever natural explanations are supplied to explain these phenomena, research (such as that reported in a ten-year study: George Meek, ed., *Healers and the Healing Process*) consistently reveals that the lowest common denominator of these practices is spirit contact and/or possession. Biblically, spiritism is a forbidden practice (Deuteronomy 18:9-12) and those who engage in these methods run not only the risk of occult bondage from spiritistic influence, but even spirit possession. Potential dangers include wrong diagnosis and a psychic transference of the physical illness to a mental or spiritual level. This can have potentially worse consequences than the original physical problem. (See our *The Facts on the Occult*, Harvest House, 1990.)

## 33. What is (medical) psychometry (radionics*)?

Medical psychometry consists of methods of psychic diagnosis and treatment. These different practices claim to work by teaching healers an alleged psychic sensitivity to "radiations" or mystical energies in objects or people. Such

---

* Radionics is a form of psychometry where the healer is aided by a mechanical apparatus such as Abram's black box or a pendulum.

sensitivity supposedly permits one to diagnose a patient's physical condition and/or prescribe treatment (e.g., use of radionics devices or homeopathic remedies). Homeopathy frequently employs these methods, and water dowsing and other forms of dowsing are forms of radionics practice claiming a natural sensitivity to water or various "radiations."

These methods have never been proven to work as claimed. For example, it is scientifically proven that radionic devices such as dowsing rods contain no mysterious powers in themselves (see Question 16). These techniques operate through spiritistic power, not a natural human or mechanical sensitivity to strange "radiations." Psychic development is required for their use and their practices are basically forms of spiritistic, psychic diagnosis and healing (see Question 32).

Potential problems include incorrect diagnosis of a serious illness, wrong prescribing of treatment, and occultic influence as revealed in such texts as *Spirit Psychometry*.

### 34. What is psychosynthesis?

Psychosynthesis is a psychological/occultic method of personal enlightenment. It was developed by psychiatrist and occultist Roberto Assagioli, a colleague of both Freud and Jung, as well as a pioneering psychotherapist in Italy. Assagioli studied Eastern and Western philosophy and the occult, and was for a number of years the Italian director of the occult movement founded by New Age leader Alice Bailey, the Arcana/Lucis Trust.

The purpose of psychosynthesis is to establish contact with an alleged inner "higher self" to receive its supposed wisdom and inspiration. In order to achieve contact and harmony with the higher self, varieties of New Age methods are employed. For example, some techniques include guided imagery, meditation, development of the will, Jungian psychology, dream work, Eastern meditation, Gestalt therapy, visualization, development of intuition, and psychodrama.

As a result of his occultic studies, Assagioli believed that every individual has seven "layers" of consciousness; the purpose of psychosynthesis is a complete integration of these seven states of consciousness. Because psychosynthesis was developed by an occultist who incorporated occultic theories and practices into his method, psychosynthesis may become the means to secure occult goals. For example, contact with one's alleged "higher self," "collective unconscious," etc., can be a disguise for contact with a spirit entity who masquerades as a psychological dynamic. Assagiolo himself believed that the "higher self" knew the future and would personally guide an individual.

Unfortunately, when the goal of therapy is to contact an inner source of wisdom, to establish dialogue with it, and to receive its teachings, the method becomes a potential means to spiritistic contact and inspiration.

### 35. What is reflexology?

Reflexology is a novel form of acupressure employing foot or hand massage. Reflexology claims to work by manipulating life-energies (*chi, prana*) through specific foot and hand massage, claiming that such massage breaks up so-called crystalline deposits that presumably obstruct *pranic* energy flow. When the flow is restored, it reaches bodily organs and systems, bringing health.

In reality, foot or hand massage offers none of the pretentious medical claims made by reflexologists. At best, reflexology gives a good massage. At worst, it can be a form of psychic development and energy channeling. Medically, it is useless.

### 36. What is Reiki?

Reiki is an ancient Japanese technique which stresses psychic healing through the manipulation of mystical life-energies. Reiki was "rediscovered" in Japan by Dr. Mikaousui in the mid-1800s. Allegedly, after many years of studying ancient Indian writings, he invented a formula for activating and directing mystical life-energy.

Reiki is a process designed not only for psychic healing, but for personal spiritual (occult) transformation as well. In order to become a Reiki instructor, one must be initiated by one of the Reiki "masters." During the process of learning the technique, the master injects psychic energy into the student, allegedly opening his psychic centers (*chakras*) and activating his "life force." This process is reminiscent of the Eastern gurus' dramatic transmission of occult power into disciples known as *shaktipat diksha*. It may also be used to assist people in entering "higher" states of consciousness.

For example, initiation for the First Reiki Degree includes four specific "attunements." These secret and solemn ceremonies permit the master to activate the universal life-force in the student. This allegedly enables the initiate to receive and then channel psychic energy. In the Second

Reiki Degree, the initiate progresses into absent healing (the psychic healing of individuals at a distance).

Reiki is thus an occult technique designed to manipulate occultic energies. Reiki instructors function in a manner indistinguishable from psychic healers who utilize spirit guides.

In Reiki we find the same problem illustrated through therapeutic touch, polarity therapy, and similar methods. The practice appears innocent and many people assume it "can't hurt." Unfortunately, occult practices can and do harm and they are anything but innocent.

### 37. What is self-help therapy?

Self-help therapy is an umbrella term for dozens of practices which employ supposed mystical inner processes as personal healers. These practices involve turning inward to seek the alleged "health wisdom" of inner guides, "sanctified" imagination, Jungian "archetypes," etc. Concepts from Jungian psychology in particular are employed in these practices. The basic assumption is that every person has a divine "inner core" or "higher self" which can be contacted by the proper methods (meditation, visualization, shamanistic practices, etc.). This mystical core is a reservoir of wisdom and information on any number of subjects including health and healing.

The basic problem with self-help therapy (e.g., using inner guides and imagination as personal healers) is the reliance on an alleged divine inner nature. Biblically, the inner nature of man is not divine nor is it a storehouse of divine wisdom; rather man's true nature is sinful and self-serving (Jeremiah 17:9; Matthew 15:19,20).

Unfortunately, self-help therapy is frequently spiritism masked under neutral terminology and redefined as latent human potential. Possible hazards include occultic influences and problems related to an attempted self-healing of serious illness (see Question 42).

### 38. What is shamanistic medicine?

Shamanistic medicine* is the application of animistic and various ancient witchcraft techniques to health care. It may involve either shamanism itself as a means to health and enlightenment (shaman initiation and following the

---

* A shaman is a pagan priest who has acquired occult powers through spirit possession.

shaman's "life path"), or the varied use of specific shamanistic techniques in conjunction with a particular health
program (visualization, altered states of consciousness,
dream work, use of "power animals" [spirits that appear in
the form of animals, birds, or other creatures to instruct the
shaman], etc.).

Shamanistic medicine claims that its methods will bring
healing for a wide variety of physical and psychological
problems and also that it will bring a practitioner into
harmony with nature, thereby maintaining health.

Because shamanism is an occult path claiming contact
with supernatural entities, it is not a legitimate medical
practice, but rather a form of ancient spiritism. Shamans
are, by definition, spirit-possessed individuals whose lives
are regulated by their spirit guides. In fact, achieving true
health according to shamanism demands that the practitioner be "energized" by his/her "power animal" or spirit
guide. Thus, healing and possession by spirits are one and
the same. In shamanism, possession by one or more spirits
for empowerment, personal health maintenance, and healing abilities is fundamental. Because the shaman himself is
spirit possessed, those individuals whom he treats run the
risk of spirit influence or even possession themselves.

It should be noted that using shamanistic techniques in
a health program is not necessarily the same thing as
following the shamanic path. One may lead to the other, but
they are not equivalent. Shamanic methods may introduce
one to shamanism which may or may not lead to pursuing
the life-path of the shaman. Nevertheless, the potential
dangers of shamanistic practice include temporary insanity, demon possession, extreme physical suffering from
shaman initiation, and conversion to occultism as a result of
being treated with shamanic techniques.

## 39. What is subliminal programming?

The audio and audio-visual self-help industry is a multi-
billion dollar enterprise. People everywhere pay hundreds
of dollars for instructional materials on buying and selling
real estate, weight loss, improving self-image, bettering
school performance, etc.

Many instructional tapes are helpful, offering straight-
forward learning sessions. Others employ the principle that
repetition of common sense guidelines for living help inte-
grate sound thinking patterns into one's life—much in the
same way Scripture memorization does.

But audio/visual tapes that are used for questionable or
occultic purposes also exist and should be avoided. For

example, many tapes make false claims or encourage visualization to experience altered states of consciousness or out-of-body experiences. Tapes that make false claims, are unrealistic, or promote a personal self-image based on distortions are not likely to be helpful.

Secular and Christian "subliminal" tapes are an example. The *Oxford American Dictionary* defines subliminal as "below the threshold of consciousness," as in advertising that seeks to influence a viewer without his conscious perception. The widely heralded claims as to the effectiveness of subliminal tapes are questionable at best. In 1990, *Psychology And Marketing* devoted two special issues to the subject, noting that ineffectiveness and fraud were evident. Because subliminal messages cannot be heard by normal means, unreputable promoters can easily sell bogus tapes and make large profits. Nevertheless, even when messages are present, those who have independently researched the claims for subliminal programming have concluded that there is no evidence that subliminal messages can influence motivation or complex behavior.

### 40. What is therapeutic touch?

Therapeutic touch is a form of psychic healing stressing the manipulation of alleged body energies such as *prana*.

Therapeutic touch was developed by two psychics, Dolores Krieger and Dora Kunz; Kunz is the current president of the occultic Theosophical Society. Therapeutic touch claims to work by channeling (psychic transfer) of the therapist's supposed *prana* (mystical energy) into the patient. Practitioners claim that this prods the patient's own "life energies" toward healing.

Therapeutic touch appears so innocent and is sufficiently accepted within the nursing profession that many people refuse to classify it as a form of psychic healing. But this is exactly what it is. Therapeutic touch: (1) was developed by psychic healers; (2) requires altered states of consciousness; (3) develops psychic ability; and (4) utilizes other occultic activity such as dowsing (see Question 16), and may be associated with other occult practices. Further, users' descriptions of their practice are indistinguishable from those of psychic healers, and recommended teaching strategies for learning therapeutic touch include books by psychic healers, mediums, and other spiritists. Because the power behind psychic healing is spiritistic, the same conclusion holds true for therapeutic touch. Unfortunately, practices like this are increasing the acceptance of psychic healing in our hospitals. We may soon reach English standards where thousands of mediums are free to operate within hospitals. The potential hazards of all such methods include incorrect diagnosis and treatment and occultic influence.

### 41. What is Touch for Health?

Touch for Health is the evaluation of a patient's condition by testing the alleged strength or weakness of muscles. It is a popularized presentation of George Goodhart's applied kinesiology (see Question 27).

Developed by chiropractor John Thie, the practice claims that body organs and systems are related to particular muscles through the alleged meridian system. The muscles that test "weak" indicate a blockage of "life energy" (*chi*) to the corresponding organ. By acupressure (finger pressure on acupuncture points), hand passes (tracing meridian lines over the body), or other methods, the flow of *chi* is allegedly restored, muscles restrengthened, and body organs and systems reinvigorated.

However, muscles are not related to organ systems in the manner that Touch for Health claims, making such diagnosis and treatment useless. Further, this practice can potentially become a form of psychic diagnosis and healing. Touch for Health may not only involve one in occultic influences, but a patient may draw false conclusions concerning the state of his/her overall health, as in alleged food allergies or other medical conditions supposedly determined to exist.

### 42. What is visualization?

New Age visualization is the use of mental concentration and directed imagery in the attempt to secure particular physical, mental, or spiritual (occult) goals. The practice of visualization is ancient and claims to work in a variety of ways. For example, by using the mind to contact an alleged inner divinity or "higher self," practitioners claim they can manipulate their personal reality to secure desired goals such as optimum health and the acquisition of wealth.

Scientific research on forms of imagery (not necessarily visualization) has provided useful insights into brain/mind interaction and the ability of mental processes to sometimes affect mind-body function. Unfortunately, modern science does not always employ proper guidelines to separate legitimate and questionable research. Such research is easily misused when tied to parapsychological/New Age premises or goals.

Visualization is often used as a means to or in conjunction with altered states of consciousness and it is often accompanied by occultic meditation. It has long been associated with pagan religion and practice such as shamanism and shamanistic medicine. It is frequently used to develop psychic abilities and in channeling to contact "inner advisers" or spirit guides. Many occultic New Age seminars such as Silva Mind Control (with seven million graduates) and est/The Forum (with one million graduates) employ it in their programs.

The basic problem is that New Age visualization assigns the human mind a divine or nearly divine status. This not only represents a major distortion of human nature, it may also mask spiritistic manipulation of the mind, defining the process as a natural or divine endeavor.

The use of visualization in health practice can lead to occultic influences and problems arising from the denial of reality by overreliance upon one's "divine" mind and its alleged healing power or health "wisdom." In the field of medicine (physical self-diagnosis) and religion (psychic revelation), the process can produce a trust in false data that could result in physical damage or spiritual deception.

### 43. What is yoga?

Millions of people employ yoga as an alleged health exercise or as part of a broader program of health maintenance. But true yoga is the occult use of breathing exercises (see Question 11), physical postures, and meditation (see Question 26) for supposed spiritual enlightenment. One of the major developers was Patanjali (ca. 400 A.D.), the compiler of the classical Raja yoga text *Yogasutra*.

The physical exercises of yoga are believed to prevent disease and maintain health through bodily regulation of *prana* (mystical energy). Further, because the body is viewed as a crude layer of the mind (see Question 10), various manipulations of the physical body (some severe) can allegedly affect the mind, bringing supposed spiritual (occult) enlightenment.

In Hindu mythology, the serpent goddess Kundalini "rests" at the base of the spine. She is aroused by yoga practice, travels up the spine regulating *prana*, opens the body's alleged *chakras* (psychic centers), unleashes psychic powers, and finally reaches the top or crown *chakra* permitting occult enlightenment. Symptoms of kundalini arousal—

which frequently constitutes spirit possession—include indescribable mental and physical pain, undiagnosable medical conditions (some severe), and/or temporary and sometimes permanent insanity.

Different Eastern or mystical religions practice different forms of yoga. Even in a given religion, there are various schools depending on the emphasis. In Hinduism, we find Hatha (physical), Raja (mental), Bhakti (devotional or emotional), Jana (knowledge or spiritual), Siddha (psychic powers), Karma (action or social responsibility), Laya (sound), Mantra, and other yogas. Kundalini may be labeled as a separate yoga; however, it should be observed that *all* yoga may arouse kundalini. Although the emphasis may vary, the basic goal is similar: union with ultimate reality, however defined. In Hinduism this would be union of the individual self (*atman*) with the supreme self (*paramatman*), itself one with Brahman, the highest impersonal Hindu god. In Buddhism it would incorporate union with *nirvana*, etc. Whatever its goal, yoga is characteristically a pagan, occultic practice.

The problems presented by yoga are both individual and social. Widespread claims to the contrary, it is *not* a health practice. The person who engages in yoga for health purposes may find himself converted to an occultic way of life. In spite of its perception as a safe and valuable technique, true yoga involves occultic meditation and the development of psychic powers which may result in spirit contact or spirit possession.

Although the public falsely perceives yoga as a safe or neutral practice, even authoritative yoga literature is replete with warnings of serious physical consequences, mental derangement, and harmful spiritual effects. Paralysis, insanity, and death are frequently mentioned. Allegedly, such consequences arise from *wrong* yoga practice but, in fact, they really arise because yoga is an *occult* practice. Those who care about their overall health should not practice yoga.

# Conclusion

The New Medicine claims to offer people optimum health—physical, mental, and spiritual. However, because the methods offered are characteristically unsound and/or occultic, they are more likely to harm than to help. People who use these practices for curing disease often become victims of health fraud or converts to occultism. New Age medicine is correct in recognizing a spiritual dimension to life and health. However, the spiritual dimension it offers is a dangerous one with more potential consequences than most illnesses.

Unfortunately, whatever our current state of health, in the end, each of us will die of some illness that for us has become incurable. All of us will face death in a very personal way. But we spend so much time seeking for meaning and health in this life, we often forget about the realities of death and eternity.

Those who are searching for truth should consider the teachings of the One who claimed, "I am the truth" and "He who believes in me will live, even though he dies" (John 14:6; 11:25).

# *RECOMMENDED READING*

Position papers etc., on chiropractic, acupuncture, homeopathy, and other treatments, from the National Council Against Health Fraud, Box 1276, Loma Linda, CA 92354, (714) 824-4690. Materials list available from NCAHF Resource Center, 3521 Broadway, Kansas City, MO 64111, (816) 753-8850).

Cover story, "The Promotion Has Gone High-Tech.: The Results Haven't," *Medical World News*, May 11, 1987.

John Ankerberg, *Can You Trust Your Doctor?* Wolgemuth & Hyatt.

John Ankerberg, *The Facts on the Occult*, Harvest House.

Marlin Y. Nelson, "Health Professionals and Unproven Medical Alternatives," *Journal of Pharmacy Technology*, March/April 1988.

Douglas Stalker, Clark Glymour, eds., *Examining Holistic Medicine*, Prometheus Books.

Petr Skrabanek, James McCormick, *Follies and Fallacies in Medicine*, Prometheus Books.

David and Sharon Sneed, *The Hidden Agenda: A Critical View of Alternative Medical Therapies*, Thomas Nelson.

Samuel Pfeifer, *Healing at Any Price?*, Milton Keynes, England: Word Limited.

Paul Reisser, *New Age Medicine*, InverVarsity.

Merril Unger, *Biblical Demonology*, Scripture Press, and *Demons in the World Today*, Tyndale.

Kurt Koch, *Christian Counseling and Occultism*, Kregel, and *Demonology: Past and Present*, Kregel.